OLIVE LEAF EXTRACT

The Mediterranean *Healing* Herb

Lori Barrett

live healthy now!

HEALTHY LIVING PUBLICATIONS
Summertown, Tennessee

Editor: Jo Stepaniak
Cover and interior design: Scattaregia Design

Healthy Living Publications,
a division of Book Publishing Company
PO Box 99
Summertown, TN 38483
888-260-8458
bookpubco.com

ISBN: 978-1-57067-333-7

Printed in the United States of America

20 19 18 17 16 15 1 2 3 4 5 6 7 8 9

Library of Congress Cataloging-in-Publication Data is available upon request.

Printed on recycled paper

Book Publishing Company is a member of Green Press Initiative. We chose to print this title on paper with 100% post-consumer recycled content, processed without chlorine, which saved the following natural resources:

- 18 trees
- 563 pounds of solid waste
- 8,414 gallons of water
- 1,551 pounds of greenhouse gases
- 8 million BTUs of energy

For more information on Green Press Initiative, visit greenpressinitiative.org. Environmental impact estimates were made using the Environmental Defense Fund Paper Calculator. For more information, visit papercalculator.org.

CONTENTS

Introduction

Americans have been stocking their kitchens with olive oil since the 1980s, when researchers first proclaimed the health benefits of a Mediterranean diet. Even before the start of the twenty-first century, when celebrities and television chefs began sprinkling extra-virgin olive oil in their skillets and over their salads, sales of olive oil soared.

The olive tree has more to offer than just its fruit, which is something alternative health practitioners have known for years. The leaves and bark are remarkably resistant to disease and drought, allowing some trees to live up to an impressive five hundred years or longer. Italy, Greece, Lebanon, Israel, and Palestine each have claimed the world's oldest olive tree. Indeed, these countries are home to gnarled, thousand-year-old olive trees. Because of these impressive life spans, scientists have tried to determine what properties give the trees their hardiness. They've discovered that olive leaves have the healthful benefits of the fruit and the disease resistance of the tree.

The Bible refers to the olive tree as "the tree of life," and it is filled with numerous references to olive trees and olive oil. During biblical times, olive oil was an important commodity and had a wide range of uses, from food to skin care to ceremonial purposes to religious rites.

Olive trees were cherished not only for their oil and fruit but also for the silver-green leaves they produced. The chemical makeup of olive leaves can vary, depending on where the trees are grown and the cultivar of the tree. Although native to the Mediterranean region, olive trees are now cultivated around the globe. In the United States, California has become a serious contender in the olive oil market. Other states, including Arizona, Georgia, and Texas, produce smaller batches of olive oils.

Unless the trees are ornamental, the leaves contain phenolic compounds that have antioxidant effects. In the regions where olive trees are native, the leaves have been used medicinally for centuries. In the 1800s, they were used to fight malaria. Olive leaf tea was made in Italy for hundreds of years, especially in Abruzzo, where it was prized for its health-enhancing qualities. Even today olive leaf tea remains a vibrant part of traditional Italian folk remedies.

Both olives and olive leaves contain the chemical compound oleuropein. Oleuropein is believed to have strong medicinal properties as an antibacterial, antibiotic, antifungal, and antiviral agent. The compound is also thought to help increase the body's immune response. Oleuropein contributes to the slightly bitter taste of olives and olive oil. Once the olives reach maturity, though, the level of oleuropein they contain declines. Even more oleuropein is lost when olives are cured. However, this is not the case with the leaves.

Oleuropein was first isolated from olive leaves in the early 1900s. It was then thought that it was the compound that helped olive trees resist disease, and scientists hoped it would have the same effect on human ailments. In the latter part of the twentieth century, research conducted on the compound found that it decreased blood pressure in laboratory animals, and it was then that the compound came into widespread use as a supplement.

Phytochemicals

"Phytochemicals" is the umbrella term for a broad category of biologically active chemical compounds found in fruits, vegetables, grains, and other plant foods. These compounds have healthful properties that are linked to a reduction in the risk of major chronic diseases. Phytochemicals are what give plant foods their color, aroma, flavor, and natural disease resistance. More than six thousand phytochemicals have been identified, but it's estimated that a large percentage still remain unknown and only a small fraction have been studied closely.

Our bodies are regularly confronted by a number of threats—just like the olive tree—from surprise infections or viruses to chronic conditions, such as arthritis, diabetes, hypertension, and inflammation. There's a common culprit among many of these ailments: destructive cells called free radicals. Free radicals are molecules with unpaired electrons. Normally, bonds don't split in a way that leaves a molecule with an unpaired electron. But when weak bonds split, free radicals are formed. Free radicals are very unstable and react quickly with other compounds, trying to capture the needed electron to gain stability. Generally, free radicals attack the nearest stable molecule, "stealing" its electron. When the molecule that is "attacked" loses its electron, it becomes a free radical itself, beginning a chain reaction. Once the process is started, it can cascade, ultimately resulting in the disruption of a living cell.

Some free radicals are created normally during the process of metabolism. Sometimes cells from the body's immune system intentionally create free radicals to neutralize viruses and bacteria. However, environmental factors, such as pollution, radiation, cigarette smoke, pesticides, and herbicides, can also generate free radicals.

Normally the body can handle free radicals, but if antioxidants (substances that fight free radicals and combat oxidative stress) are unavailable, or if the free-radical production becomes excessive, damage can occur. It is particularly noteworthy that free-radical damage accumulates with age. Because oxidative stress induced by free radicals is associated with a wide range of chronic diseases, and because phytochemicals are antioxidants, it's possible that the health benefits of phytochemicals in fruits and vegetables may be even greater than what is currently understood.

Phytochemical Concentrations in Food

Although color is a good indicator of phytochemical content, it's just one useful measure, as some phytochemicals are colorless, and one color might mask another color. Foods in a particular color group will have varying amounts of the same phytochemical. In addition, some phytochemicals are responsible for how a food tastes.

Phytochemicals are found in all edible parts of a fruit or vegetable, but they are most concentrated in the skin. Both genetics and environmental factors can greatly affect the amount of phytochemicals a food contains. Some of the most important environmental influences on phytochemical concentrations in food include the following:

- Altitude
- Climate
- Temperature
- Sunlight exposure
- Soil composition
- Irrigation
- Maturity of the plant
- Predation exposure (attacks by bacteria, molds, or insects will increase phytochemical content as the plant tries to fight off the attacker)
- Storage conditions
- Processing and preparation methods

Types of Phytochemicals

Scientists group phytochemicals according to their chemical structure. This often means that phytochemicals in a group act in the human body in a similar way. Two broad classes of phytochemicals that most people are familiar with are flavonoids and carotenoids.

Most fruits and vegetables can be classified into one of five color groups: blue/purple, green, red, white, and yellow/orange. When we eat broadly from each of these groups every day, we're assured of obtaining a wide range of phytochemicals. The following table shows the various phytochemicals found in each color group:

Phytochemicals by color

Color	Flavonoids	Carotenoids	Other Phyto-chemicals
Blue/purple	Anthocyanidins Flavan-3-ols Flavonols Proanthocyanidins		Ellagic acid Resveratrol
Green	Flavanones Flavones Flavonols	Beta-carotene Lutein Zeaxanthin	Indols Isothiocyanates Organosulfur compounds
Red	Anthocyanidins Flavan-3-ols Flavanones Flavones Flavonols Proanthocyanidins	Lycopene	Ellagic acid Resveratrol
White	Flavanones Flavonols		Indols Isothiocyanates Organosulfur compounds
Yellow/orange	Flavanones Flavonols	Alpha-carotene Beta-carotene Beta-cryptoxanthin	

Source: Produce for Better Health Foundation, Phytochemical Info Center (pbhfoundation.org), May 2015.

Flavonoids

Flavonoids, also called bioflavonoids, are the largest, most varied, and most studied group of phytochemicals. They are perhaps best known for their rich diversity of color-providing plant pigments, such as the deep blue of blueberries, the dark purple of grapes, and the vibrant red of cranberries. The word derives from the Latin term *flavus*, meaning "yellow." Flavonoids are among the largest nutrient families, with thousands of unique flavonoids having been identified by researchers.

Dietary intakes of certain foods rich in flavonoids are associated with reduced risk of death due to coronary heart disease and cardiovascular disease. Fruits and vegetables are the main dietary sources of flavonoids for humans. There is also flavonoid data on nuts and seeds, grains, and legumes (peas, beans, and lentils), and select other foods and beverages (for example, red wine and green and black teas). However, scientists are challenged with accurately measuring the daily intake of flavonoids because of discrepancies among various food sources. Nevertheless, research on the health aspects of flavonoids is expanding rapidly, and many flavonoids have been shown to provide neurological support and to have antioxidative activity, free-radical scavenging capacity, coronary heart disease preventive capabilities, and anticancer activity.

The United States Department of Agriculture's Flavonoid Database breaks down its flavonoid analyses into five of the basic flavonoid chemical subgroups:

1. anthocyanidins (such as cyanidin, delphinidin, malvidin, pelargonidin, peonidin, and petunidin).
2. flavan-3-ols (such as catechins, epicatechins, gallocatechins, and theaflavins)
3. flavones (such as apigenin and luteolin)
4. flavonols (such as isorhamnetin, kaempferol, myricetin, and quercetin)
5. flavanones (such as eriodictyol, hesperetin, and naringenin)

As shown in the table below, it takes a wide variety of foods to cover these five categories of flavonoids:

Sample food sources of flavonoids

Anthocyanidins	Flavan-3-ols	Flavones	Flavonols	Flavanones
Bananas	Apples	Apples	Almonds	Grapefruits
Cabbages	Blueberries	Cantaloupe	Chickpeas	Oranges
Cherries	Peaches	Celery	Onions	Tomatoes

Chickpeas	Pears	Chiles	Quinoa	
Cranberries	Strawberries	Lettuces	Romaine lettuce	
Pears		Oranges	Sweet potatoes	
Plums		Parsley	Tomatoes	
Raspberries			Turnip greens	
Strawberries				

Source: USDA Database for the Flavonoid Content of Selected Foods, Release 3.1 (December 2013).

In the United States, over half of all flavonoid intake comes from the flavan-3-ol category, the subgroup that is so concentrated in green and black teas. The average daily consumption of flavonoids in the United States is between 250 and 275 milligrams. Currently, there is no Dietary Reference Intake (DRI) or Daily Value (DV) for optimal flavonoid amounts, and finding accurate comprehensive information about the overall flavonoid content in foods is difficult. However, based on current dietary recommendations, if a person consumed ten servings of whole, natural fruits and vegetables per day, the total flavonoid intake would be close to 1,000 milligrams or higher. Because a disproportionate amount of the flavonoids consumed in the United States come from a single flavonoid subgroup, there is likely to be flavonoid deficiency from the other subgroups. This deficiency of flavonoids reflects the overall low dietary intake of fresh, natural fruits and vegetables in the United States, along with a high consumption of processed and overcooked foods. The best way to ensure ample flavonoid intake is to maximize dietary intake of whole natural foods, including fresh, brightly colored vegetables and fruits.

There currently is no evidence that dietary flavonoids are toxic, even in meals that contain an abundance of fresh fruits and vegetables along with other whole plant foods. In addition, because these foods are high in dietary fiber, the quantity we eat of them at a sitting is generally self-limiting. In addition, since flavonoids are water soluble, it can be assumed that they involve a lower risk of toxicity than is associated with fat-soluble nutrients.

Surprisingly, olive leaf extract contains a diverse number of flavonoids, including apigenin, chrysoeriol, hesperetin, kaempferol, luteolin, quercetin, and rutin. As a result, olive leaf extract encompasses a broad range of flavonoid subgroups simultaneously, making it easy to obtain an extensive number of phytochemicals from this single source.

Antioxidants and Health

Antioxidants and the Mediterranean Diet

Antioxidants are compounds found in whole foods that fight oxidation and help protect the body from free-radical damage. They came to public attention in the 1990s, not long after the Mediterranean diet started gaining popularity, as scientists began to figure out that damage from free radicals was linked to cancer and cardiovascular disease. It was found that in the countries bordering the Mediterranean Sea, people were living longer and suffering fewer cases of heart disease and cancer compared to people in North America. The people of the Mediterranean region had diets centered primarily on plant-based foods, such as fruits, vegetables, whole grains, legumes, and nuts. And rather than using animal fats, they used healthy fats, such as olive oil.

Research has come to show that the traditional Mediterranean diet indeed reduces the risk of heart disease. In fact, an analysis of more than 1.5 million healthy adults demonstrated that following a Mediterranean diet was associated with a reduced risk of death from heart disease and cancer, as well as a reduced incidence of Parkinson's disease and Alzheimer's disease. The Dietary Guidelines for Americans recommends the Mediterranean diet as an eating plan that can help promote health and prevent disease. Key components of the Mediterranean diet include the following:

- Eating primarily plant-based foods, such as fruits and vegetables, whole grains, legumes, and nuts
- Replacing butter with healthy fats, such as olive oil
- Using herbs and spices instead of salt to flavor foods
- Limiting or eliminating red meat and other meat
- Drinking red wine in moderation (optional)

Instead of limiting total fat consumption, the Mediterranean diet emphasizes choosing healthier types of fat and features olive oil as the primary source of fat. Olive oil is mainly monounsaturated fat—a type of fat that can help reduce LDL ("bad") cholesterol levels when used in place of saturated or trans fats. Extra-virgin and virgin olive oils are the least processed forms and also contain the highest levels of protective plant compounds that provide antioxidant effects.

Measuring Antioxidants in Foods

There is scientific evidence that the antioxidants found in whole plant foods, such as fruits, vegetables, and whole grains, work to fight diseases. But there is no evidence that individual antioxidant supplements, such as beta-carotene, vitamin C, vitamin E, or food products with artificially added antioxidant compounds are beneficial. What is certain is that antioxidants are most effective when they're consumed from their natural sources, which often contain a spectrum of antioxidants.

There are labs that aim to quantify the antioxidant properties of foods and supplements. The United States Department of Agriculture (USDA) and the National Institutes of Health developed a scale of oxygen radical absorbance capacity, known as ORAC. The USDA had an extensive database of foods based on their ORAC level, but they dismantled the database in 2012 out of concern that the specific metabolic functions of the antioxidants are unproved. Their tests measured antioxidant effects in vitro—in test tubes—but they weren't able to duplicate the results in humans.

Some health and nutrition experts believe the USDA's statements about ORAC were incorrect and misleading and have rebutted the agency's decision. Their rationale is summarized in Brunswick Laboratories' critical response to the USDA ORAC statement as outlined on their website (brunswicklabs.com) and detailed below:

1. No in vitro assay that quantifies a characteristic of a nutritional product describes in vivo outcomes and should not be used to suggest such a connection.
2. Vital information about metabolism, bioavailability, mechanisms of action, and efficacy is not measured by any such in vitro assay.
3. There is evidence that polyphenols are connected to beneficial human health outcomes.
4. There is evidence that these beneficial outcomes have antioxidant as well as diverse other mechanisms of action.
5. ORAC has been and remains a valuable analytical tool in connection with other investigative methods.

Other labs have continued to test ORAC levels of foods and supplements. The website superfoodly.com/orac-values lists the antioxidant levels of different foods and includes the following statement: "While the exact relationship between the ORAC value of a food and its health benefit has not been established, it is believed that foods higher on the ORAC scale will more effectively neutralize free radicals. According to the free-radical theory of aging, this will slow the oxidative processes and free radical damage that can contribute to age-related degeneration and disease."

In addition to the ORAC score, other tests measure antioxidant levels. One such test compares Trolox, a cell-permeable, water-soluble derivative of vitamin E with potent antioxidant properties, to other antioxidants. It's called the Trolox equivalent antioxidant capacity, or TEAC. Another test measures the ferric-reducing ability of plasma, or FRAP. And yet another measures the total radical-trapping antioxidant parameter, or TRAP. None of these tests are perfect, however. Scientists are still working on a standardized measure so when consumers see an antioxidant claim on food packaging, they'll know exactly what that number means. Even as the scientific community debates measurements, they still agree that antioxidants are a powerful weapon in the fight against disease.

Antioxidant Properties of Olive Leaves

Different manufacturers of olive leaf extract have tested their products' ORAC levels. The scores vary, but they consistently come in higher than the ORAC levels for green tea or vitamin C.

One of the most cited studies on the antioxidant properties of olive leaves comes from a group of scientists at Southern Cross University in Australia. Prompted by the prevalence of urinary and kidney disorders in industrialized societies, the scientists from the pharmacology and medicine departments tested fifty-five medicinal herbs that had been linked to traditional treatments for kidney problems. They used three different solvents to make liquid extractions, and tested the ORAC levels of the extractions. Milk thistle and tea leaf were used as comparison herbs, as both have high antioxidant capacities. The results, which were published in the *Journal of Alternative and Complementary Medicine* in February 2007, showed that twelve of the herbs were comparable to or exceeded the ORAC levels of tea leaves and milk thistle, and of those twelve, olive leaf extract had one of the highest scores.

In 2013 a team of Spanish researchers looked at the antioxidant capacity of olive leaf extract in human trials. Their study, published in the *European Journal of Nutrition,* tested oral use of olive leaf extract by premenopausal and postmenopausal women. Their results suggest that postmenopausal women could benefit from taking olive leaf extract because the antioxidant oleuropein can stave off the oxidative stress that leads to conditions such as osteoporosis.

In the 1960s, The Upjohn Company, a large pharmaceutical manufacturer at that time, determined that elenolic acid, which is derived from oleuropein, fights viruses and bacteria. The Upjohn Company created calcium elenolate, a synthetic, from the natural elenolic acid in oleuropein and pitted it against a series of viruses. The calcium elenolate inhibited growth of the viruses in test tubes, but when researchers moved on to tests with human and animal blood, the blood proteins bound to the calcium elenolate and rendered it ineffective. As a result, The Upjohn Company abandoned its testing of the olive leaf compounds. However, other scientists linked the failure of The Upjohn Company's tests to its use of synthetic compounds—the calcium elenolate they had created. Some researchers later built upon The Upjohn Company's work, using oleuropein alone and in conjunction with other natural compounds found in olive leaves. Natural health practitioners and marketers of olive leaf extract debate the role of oleuropein; some say it's one of many active ingredients in olive leaves while others say it's the ingredient that gives the leaves their potency.

The Healing Power of Olive Leaves

Around the same time that awareness of antioxidants was growing, the medical community started to acknowledge public interest in medicinal plants. Even though modern medicine has become increasingly available in developing countries, local populations still rely on herbal remedies. The World Health Organization published a guide to medicinal plants in 1999 to help provide consumers and medical professionals with scientific information on medicinal plants and their efficacy, traditional uses and dosages, and contraindications and common sensitivities. Even websites such as WebMD.com and MayoClinic.org now list herbal remedies for many conditions.

Olive leaves gained media attention in Great Britain and Australia in July 2012, when Australian swimmer James Magnussen—then the world champion in the 100-meter freestyle—drank a mix of olive leaf extract and probiotics at a press conference before a meet. In January 2013, author, educator, and "medicine hunter" Chris Kilham, who researches and promotes plant-based medicines and natural cures around the world, wrote an article about olive leaves and their use in the Mediterranean that appeared on the Fox News website. He said that even though the leaves aren't as well known as the fruit and the oil derived from the fruit, a growing body of science shows the leaves are worthy of their ancient medicinal reputation. "In the world of medicinal plants, it is often the case that traditional use of plants precedes, by centuries, the science that corroborates the same uses. This is certainly true with olive leaf," Kilham wrote.

Because olive leaves have a long history in folk medicine as a tonic or tea to treat malaria and as an antiseptic for wounds, modern science has started to pay attention. All over the world, researchers are testing the healing powers of the compounds in olive leaves. The following table lists the primary compounds in olive leaves and the health benefits attributed to them:

Main olive leaf compounds and their benefits

Compound	**Class**	**Health Benefits**
Apigenin	Flavonoid	Linked to cancer prevention
Caffeic acid	Phenolic acid	Linked to cancer prevention
Catechin	Flavonoid	Linked to cancer prevention
Hydroxytyrosol	Polyphenol	Anti-inflammatory; linked to bone health
Luteolin	Flavonoid	Linked to cancer prevention
Oleuropein	Polyphenol	Anti-inflammatory; antimicrobial; antiviral; linked to bone health
Quercetin	Flavonoid	Anti-inflammatory; antihistamine
Tyrosol	Polyphenol	Possible neuroprotective properties; linked to cancer prevention

Source: Produce for Better Health Foundation, Phytochemical Info Center (pbhfoundation.org), May 2015.

Combating Disease with Olive Leaves

Bacteria and Bacterial Infections

Although bacteria in general have developed a far-reaching bad reputation, not all bacteria are harmful. The word "bacteria" appears on a wide variety of labels, from cleaning products to yogurt, and it often makes its way into headline news. Probiotic bacteria have enjoyed an almost superhero status in recent years, partly because scientists are looking for ways to fight pathogens that have built up resistance caused by our modern overreliance on sanitizing products and antibiotics.

Michael Pollan wrote in the *New York Times* in 2013 about germs and their integral role in human health. He took part in a project that sequences a person's microbiome, or the bacteria inside an individual's body. Pollan learned that the body's colony of bacteria has a direct influence on health, perhaps an even more powerful influence than genetics. If we lose the diversity in our internal ecosystem, it could potentially predispose us to obesity and a host of chronic diseases and infections. Scientists stop short of talking about cures for diseases, but Pollan points out that during most the last century we've been engaged in a war against bacteria, as evidenced by our reliance on antibiotics and a diet that has evolved to include processed foods scrubbed of all bacteria. These behaviors are detrimental to the microbiome's well-being. To be sure, Pollan doesn't suggest that antibiotics are all bad; they're certainly valuable treatments at times and overall have helped to increase our life expectancy. But, as with any war, Pollan writes, there have been unintended consequences.

The loss of diversity in our microbiome is a growing concern because it can lead to drug-resistant bacteria. The Centers for Disease Control acknowledges that almost all bacteria have grown stronger and less responsive to antibiotic treatment. There are three ways bacteria evolve to become more invulnerable: (1) microorganisms can mutate to develop resistance; (2) they can develop an ability to neutralize the antibiotic; and

(3) they can develop an ability to filter out the antibiotic. For these reasons, health care practitioners across the globe are looking for new ways to fight bacteria that won't provoke resistance, and this has led both alternative and conventional practitioners to revisit the use of medicinal plants.

Research on olive leaf extract's bacterial interactions has so far been in vitro and not yet tested directly on humans. The evidence of its use in humans is still anecdotal but goes back hundreds of years. In the 1800s, Daniel Hanbury, a British botanist and pharmacologist, traveled to the Middle East and the Mediterranean to study and collect plants. In 1854 he published the article "Notes on the Febrifuge Properties of the Olive" in *Pharmaceutical Journal.* In the article, he recounted his treatment of fevers with a concoction made from boiled olive leaves, which he said he found to be more effective than quinine. He also cited his own research that found earlier medicinal uses of olive leaves. His notes led to further inquiry and examination, most notably the studies conducted by the The Upjohn Company in the late 1960s and the 1970s.

The early research focused on oleuropein, the major bioactive compound of the olive tree and present in high amounts in unprocessed olive fruit and leaves. Cured olives are soaked in brine to eliminate their naturally bitter taste, which is attributed to the oleuropein. More recently, food scientists observed that lactic acid bacteria, one of the main components of the olive fermentation process, inhibited some pathogens. This led to a flurry of studies and news articles in the Mediterranean touting the potential probiotic properties of olives.

The bacterial response that occurs during the fermentation process of olives has inspired scientists to investigate the way that olive compounds react with bacteria that's present in humans. In 1999 a team of researchers in Italy tested strains of bacteria for in vitro susceptibility to oleuropein and hydroxytyrosol, a polyphenol thought to be responsible for olive oil's anti-inflammatory effects. Hydroxytyrosol is a superstar among antioxidants, as it's the most powerful one discovered to date. Hydroxytyrosol has an ORAC value of 68,576, which is fifteen times higher than that of green tea and three times higher than that of CoQ10. The researchers found the hydroxytyrosol in olives to be slightly more effective against the bacterial strains than oleuropein. They surmised that these two specific olive compounds could be considered as potential sources of antimicrobial agents for treating intestinal or respiratory infections in humans.

At Technion Israel Institute of Technology, a public research university in Haifa, microbiologists tested different strains of bacteria, including *Candida albicans*, with a water extract of olive leaves. All strains of the bacteria were weakened or destroyed by the extract, although the results varied with different concentrations. The researchers concluded that their findings suggest an antimicrobial potential for olive leaves.

Cancer

Cancer extends as far back in human history as olives, yet for all the years of research and new medications, the disease remains a mystery. We know that cancer begins at the cellular level, when an abnormal cell is able to multiply or invade other tissue. The progression varies according to the type of cancer and among different people, because genetics, diet, and lifestyle can all play a part.

The timing of detection can also alter cancer's progression. If cancer is caught early on, there's a greater chance that damage can be reversed, especially if diet is factored into the treatment plan. Antioxidants and other phytochemicals work to reverse the damage caused to cells and tissues; they also can help thwart further damage. For this reason, prevention has emerged as a focus of cancer research, with a good deal of emphasis on nutrition.

Studies of regional diets have been used in the search for alternative and conventional medical treatments of disease. Links have been found between diet—in particular, fat intake—and inflammation, cancer, and coronary heart disease. These studies fall under the category of epidemiology, or the science of distribution, cause, and effect on health and disease conditions. The earliest epidemiological studies of cancer evaluated patients who were already diagnosed and compared their past diets with a control group of subjects without cancer. Newer studies start with a control group, categorized by ethnicity or geographic location. Once a group is identified, scientific trials can be conducted. Current findings are limited because only a small amount of nutrients or nutritional factors can be studied at one time.

The Harvard School of Public Health has attempted to expand on what can be learned from population studies with its Pooling Project of Prospective Studies of Diet and Cancer. The Pooling Project is an international consortium of independent groups with the goal of analyzing diet and cancer associations using standardized criteria across studies. Their objective is to evaluate whether diet and cancer associations are consistent across studies comprised of different populations with different dietary habits. They believe that their combined data will have greater precision than any individual study because of the larger sample size.

Overall, researchers agree that nutrients play a role in cancer prevention, especially when the nutrients come from whole food sources. The World Cancer Research Fund, along with the American Institute for Cancer Research, published a report in 1997 examining epidemiological research on cancer and diet factors. That report was updated in 2007, and their website (dietandcancerreport.org) provides expanded information that also includes weight and physical activity as factors, along with continuous updates. The current report carries forth the same information and advice as the original report: about one-third of all cancers are preventable with appropriate food and nutrition, regular exercise, and avoidance of obesity.

Much of modern research focuses on how specific plant compounds interact with different cancers. The American Cancer Society has acknowledged that phytochemicals play a role in the prevention and treatment of cancer, as well as diabetes, heart disease, and high blood pressure. There is even some evidence that certain phytochemicals might prevent the formation of potential carcinogens, block the action of carcinogens, or act on cells to suppress cancer development.

Another population study that examined cancer and plant nutrients focused on women in Iowa. The Iowa Women's Health Study, which originated in 1986 with two doctors from the University of Minnesota School of Public Health and the George Washington University School of Public Health, recruited more than forty-one thousand women between the ages of fifty-five and sixty-nine to participate. The purpose of the study was to determine links between diet and cancer risk and ascertain possible contributors to survival. The women were given a questionnaire at the start of the study and were then sent follow-up questionnaires over the course of several years that asked about reproductive history, medical history, risk factors, dietary intake, and physical activity. The study spawned three hundred published manuscripts based on the information compiled. Among them was a study by researchers in the Netherlands that singled out catechin, a flavonoid in green tea, black tea, cocoa, and olive leaves. The results of that study found that catechin intake may protect against rectal cancer.

Plants and plant parts have been an integral part of health care throughout history, but modern chemistry has made it possible to isolate individual compounds for study. If a compound is found to be effective in fighting disease, chemists can then work with that compound to either create a new drug or make the existing compound more digestible, soluble, or efficient in the human body. Another compound from olive leaves that has been studied in relation to cancer is apigenin.

A team of researchers from Ohio State University's Comprehensive Cancer Center found that apigenin can take away the ability of breast cancer cells to prevent their own death. Normally cancerous cells splice or modify to stay alive. The two authors of the study explained that apigenin binds with proteins in the body and influences cell behavior, particularly the cells' ability to splice. Their findings were published in the journal *Proceedings of the National Academy of the Sciences* in 2013.

Oleuropein was found to reduce skin damage from UVB irradiation. In a study using hairless mice, researchers from Ehime University School of

Medicine in Japan observed six groups of mice. Five groups were exposed to UVB irradiation. Two of the groups were treated with olive leaf extract, two of the other groups were treated with oleuropein, and the remaining group was the control. At the completion of the study, they discovered that the extract and the oleuropein prevented the increased skin thickness that accompanies sun exposure, while also preserving skin elasticity. In addition, the olive leaf extract and oleuropein decreased the incidence and growth of skin tumors.

Luteolin, another of the flavonoids in olives, olive oil, and olive leaves, has shown properties similar to those seen in oleuropein. In laboratory tests, luteolin blocked some of the signaling required for cancer cells to communicate, thereby inhibiting their growth and proliferation. A team of researchers from Korea studied colon cancer cells and found that luteolin blocked the cells' communication and ability to divide. Their research was published in BioMed Central's journal *BMC Gastroenterology* in 2012.

Because many plants with high levels of luteolin are used in traditional Chinese medicine, doctors continue to study the interaction between luteolin and cancer cells, including the way nutritional therapy might work with conventional medical therapy. Although Western medical doctors don't generally advise treating illness with plant therapies, some physicians believe that combining therapies can lead to longer survival rates, fewer side effects, and a reduced risk of disease recurrence.

Diabetes

Diabetes is a group of diseases that can develop when blood glucose levels are too high. Glucose is a major source of energy for most cells of the body, including brain cells. Carbohydrates, which are found in fruit, cereal, bread, pasta, and rice, are quickly turned into glucose in the body, raising the blood glucose level.

The hormone insulin facilitates the body's use of glucose. Type 1 diabetes is a chronic condition in which the pancreas produces insufficient or no insulin. Type 2 diabetes is a chronic condition that affects the way the body processes glucose. With type 2 diabetes, the body does not use insulin properly; this is known as insulin resistance. Initially, the pancreas makes extra insulin to make up for the improperly used insulin, but over time it can't make enough insulin to maintain normal levels, and glucose builds up in the bloodstream. Type 2 is the most common form of diabetes. The risk of developing type 2 diabetes increases with obesity because fatty tissue hinders the body's ability to process sugars. An inactive lifestyle also increases the risk of diabetes because activity helps to use up glucose.

A group of researchers in New Zealand looked at the number of people using complementary or alternative treatments for diabetes, along with the fact that studies were starting to emerge on the medicinal properties of olive products. They tested olive leaf polyphenols on humans, prompted by the history of folk use of olive leaves. The study was published in *PLOS ONE*, the journal of the Public Library of Science. The researchers started with the knowledge that about one-third of patients in Britain with type 2 diabetes use alternative medicine to manage the disease, even though there's little to no scientific proof that alternative therapies work. They recruited forty-six overweight men and conducted double-blind, randomized tests in which they gave the men olive leaf extract or placebo capsules for twelve weeks. The results showed that the oleuropein and hydroxytyrosol from the olive leaf extract improved insulin sensitivity. The outcomes were comparable to results seen with metformin, a widely prescribed diabetes medication.

Fungal Infections

Once thought to be plants, fungi are now their own kingdom of organisms. Most fungi are harmless: we eat them in the form of mushrooms or as yeast in bread, and we drink the bubbles they make in beer or champagne. They're also the basis for a class of antibiotics. Fungi reproduce by spreading spores that we breathe in or touch, and they thrive in places that have a warm, moist environment. Sometimes we pick up a fungus in the form of athlete's foot, fingernail or toenail infections, eye infections, or *Candida albicans*, which infects the mouth, throat, stomach, or urinary tract. Fungal infections are usually easy to treat, but when fungi invade tissue, they can cause serious illness, especially for people with compromised immune systems.

Normally the body has defenses against fungal invaders in the stomach and the urinary tract, but antibiotics weaken the helpful bacteria that naturally fight off fungi, making the body more susceptible to fungal infections. Generally, fungal infections don't have to be treated with antibiotics; the infection will usually just resolve on its own.

For people with weakened immune systems, however, fungal infections require medical treatment. Nevertheless, not all the treatments offered are effective, and some have annoying or serious side effects. Sometimes the body will adapt to the fungus rather than banishing it. In addition, fungi exhibit some adaptability of their own. Usually this means the fungi change in ways that will allow them to thrive in the body's acidic environment. Researchers are increasingly investigating the ways fungi adapt so they can better identify and treat fungal infections. At the same time, alternative health practitioners, and even some conventional medical doctors, recommend olive leaf extract as a treatment.

Histoplasmosis is a fungus that grows as a mold in the soil. It can make people sick with flulike symptoms when they breathe in spores produced by the fungus. Soil that contains bird or bat droppings may have larger amounts of this fungus, and the threat is greater in caves, where bats may reside, or in torn-down old buildings. Infection from histoplasmosis can occur in people with a healthy immune system, but having a weakened immune system increases the risk of getting or reactivating this disease. Very young or very old people, or those with AIDS, cancer, or an organ transplant, will experience more severe symptoms. On its website, the University of Maryland Medical Center lists olive leaf extract among its recommended herbal treatments for fungal activity, specifically histoplasmosis, and immunity. The center also suggests preparing a tea from olives leaves.

Candida is a fungus that normally exists in the mouth and intestines. It can grow out of control after a round of antibiotics or because of high stress levels or a diet high in processed foods and refined sugars. Symptoms of candida include fatigue, headaches, itchy patches on the skin, weight loss or weight gain, and nail infections, usually of the toenails. Because symptoms vary so widely, the illness is still somewhat of a mystery. Many physicians won't diagnose patients with having a *Candida albicans* infection, as they consider "candida" a catchall term rather than a specific illness. Instead, they'll treat the fatigue or headaches or rash. If candida is diagnosed, treatment usually involves a combination of antifungal medication, probiotics, and a change in diet to eliminate sugars and processed foods.

Carol Kumamoto, a professor of molecular biology and microbiology at Tufts University, has a research lab solely devoted to understanding candida. She became captivated by candida's transition point, the mysterious apex where it transforms from being harmless into being harmful. One focus of Kumamoto's research has been candida's relationship to inflammation. Kumamoto's own research, and her examination of other studies, has led her to conclude that there is a connection between a fungal invasion of the intestinal tract and inflammation; it appears that each condition worsens the other. "These effects may create a vicious cycle in which low-level inflammation promotes fungal colonization and fungal colonization promotes further inflammation," Kumamoto wrote in the journal *Current Opinion in Microbiology.*

Because it has proved effective as an anti-inflammatory, olive leaf extract is also recommended as a natural remedy for fungal infections. In *The Complete Candida Yeast Guidebook*, the authors recommend olive leaf extract as a natural antifungal. They cite research from The Upjohn Company from the 1970s that showed in in vitro studies, calcium elenolate, created from the natural elenolic acid in oleuropein, was lethal to every virus the researchers tested it against. More recent studies have demonstrated that the components of olive leaf extract are also toxic to a wide range of bacteria, parasites, protozoa, fungi, and yeasts.

Heart Health

Ideas about diet and cardiovascular health changed significantly in the 1980s, when the world first took notice of the Mediterranean diet. Ancel Keys, a University of Minnesota public health scientist who invented the pocket-sized food for soldiers known as K rations, discovered that saturated fat was a major cause of heart disease and championed the benefits of the Mediterranean diet. But as early as 1958, Keys had begun studying the eating patterns of healthy, middle-aged men in seven countries: Greece, Finland, Italy, Japan, the Netherlands, the United States, and Yugoslavia. Known as the Seven Countries Study, it was the first major study to investigate diet and lifestyle along with other risk factors for cardiovascular disease. The study involved contrasting countries and cultures and spanned an extended period of time.

Keys's results showed that people in Greece and southern Italy, who had diets rich in olives, olive oil, fruits, and vegetables and lower in animal-based foods compared with the other countries and regions, lived longer and had fewer cases of heart disease. This lent credence to the theory that a diet heavy in saturated animal fats leads to higher rates of coronary disease. The fats from olive oil didn't have the same effect on heart health as did the animal-based fats. The study also underscored the importance of maintaining a healthy weight and an active lifestyle. Keys wrote a book about the study's findings called *How to Eat Well and Stay Well the Mediterranean Way*, which was a best seller in 1975.

The Seven Countries Study was a pioneering endeavor that influenced and enhanced many studies to follow. Ancel Keys and his Italian colleague Flaminio Fidanza and their colleagues in the study were central to the modern recognition, definition, and promotion of the eating patterns they found in Italy and Greece, now popularized as "the Mediterranean diet." They demonstrated that dietary patterns in the Mediterranean at the time of the study were associated with low rates of coronary heart disease and mortality due to all causes. Studies of the elderly showed that a healthy diet and lifestyle, including getting sufficient physical activity, abstaining from smoking, and limiting alcohol consumption, were also associated with a lower risk of cardiovascular disease and general mortality.

In the years following the Seven Countries Study, other institutions and researchers set out to prove Keys's theories. Beginning in 2003, doctors at the University of Barcelona recruited more than seven thousand people who were overweight, smoked, or had other risk factors for heart disease. The participants were assigned a Mediterranean diet or a low-fat diet. This study had more controls than the Seven Countries Study, and participants were followed more closely. The participants' urine was regularly tested to ensure they adhered to their diets. Half the people on the Mediterranean diet were prescribed a specific amount of extra-virgin olive oil per day; the other half were prescribed a specific amount of tree nuts per day. After five years, the researchers concluded that the participants on the Mediterranean diet showed a significant reduction in their risk of cardiovascular problems.

Michael Aviram is a distinguished scientist who has been revolutionizing cardiovascular medicine for over three decades. A nutrition researcher and professor of biochemistry at Technion Israel Institute of Technology and head of its Lipid Research Laboratory, Aviram recommends a diet based on the seven species mentioned in the Bible: barley, date honey (a dark, sweet, thick syrup made from dates), figs, grapes, olives, pomegranates, and wheat. In addition, he states that the most cardio-protective foods overall are olive oil, pomegranates, red wine, and licorice root. Aviram's findings about the antioxidants in these ancient foods has led to some of the current research regarding olive polyphenols and cardiovascular health.

Aviram points out that there is a lot of crossover between the seven-species diet he recommends and the Mediterranean diet, but he adds that the similarities aren't just about the food choices. In ancient times people in these regions ate according to the seasons, and their food came from plants or animals directly, without first being processed in a manufacturing facility. People carved out time for meals with friends and family, they walked more, and they benefited from the mild climate. He contends that all these factors, along with the right food choices, play a part in cardiovascular health.

People with high blood pressure have a greater risk of coronary heart disease. According to the World Heart Federation, high blood pressure is the second-highest risk factor for stroke. As early as the 1950s and 1960s, researchers had begun studying the hypotensive (ability to lower blood pressure) effects of olive leaves.

In 2008, Swiss researchers tested olive leaf extract on humans, since it had been shown effective in laboratory rats. They selected forty pairs of identical twins to include in the study. Each set of twins was assigned to a different group, with one group receiving 500 milligrams of olive leaf extract per day and the other group receiving 1,000 milligrams per day. After eight weeks, the group that had received the higher dose of olive leaf extract had significantly lower blood pressure; in addition, that group had lower cholesterol.

Doctors from the University of Durban-Westville in South Africa evaluated the active compounds in local wild olive leaves, because preliminary analysis showed the local leaves to have a lesser concentration of oleuropein compared to European plants. The experiment included Greek olive leaves, Cape Town olive leaves, and African wild olive leaves. All three types of leaves proved successful at preventing high blood pressure, especially in cases where the condition was related to salt sensitivity, as well as atherosclerosis (plaque buildup in the arteries).

Inflammation

There are a variety of ways the body protects us from invasive pathogens and the injuries they can cause. As a protective barrier, our skin provides the first level of defense. The mucus in our respiratory systems and stomachs carries contaminants away. And the lymphatic organs, which include bone marrow, lymph nodes, and the spleen, thymus, and tonsils, do the heavy lifting for our immune system by transporting white blood cells as they seek and fight harmful organisms. As the white blood cells attack the invaders, the body experiences inflammation, which can be seen and felt in the resulting redness, swelling, pain, and heat. This type of inflammation is a normal part of the body's natural defense mechanisms. However, when the body experiences inflammation that's not in response to pathogens or injury, it results in harm to tissues. Chronic, persistent, misdirected inflammation can lead to Alzheimer's disease, cancer, heart disease, and rheumatoid arthritis. Because of the close link between chronic inflammation and these serious conditions, the medical community has begun researching preventive measures and cures, including the use of olive leaf extract.

At Kinki University in Osaka, Japan, researchers curious about the anti-inflammatory effects of hydroxytyrosol in olive leaf extract conducted a clinical trial with patients with gonarthrosis, a disorder of the knee joint. The patients were given hydroxytyrosol or a placebo over a period of four weeks. The group given the hydroxytyrosol showed improvement in the pain measurement index compared with the placebo group.

In the Mediterranean, olive leaves and their extracts have long been used in folk remedies for arthritis. Current scientific research has demonstrated that olive leaf extract can impede the development of several kinds of arthritis, including gout, osteoarthritis, and rheumatoid arthritis. Gout is caused by the accumulation of uric acid crystals in joints, the by-products of impaired recycling of DNA and RNA in cells. The standard drug therapy for gout is allopurinol, which often causes a number of side effects. However, oleuropein can effectively prevent the buildup of uric acid in the same way that allopurinol does, by inhibiting the enzyme responsible for converting DNA and RNA into uric acid, but without causing the unpleasant side effects associated with the drug.

Oleuropein has also been shown to benefit osteoarthritis and rheumatoid arthritis. In animal models, olive leaf extract relieved joint swelling, improved the microscopic appearance of joint tissue, and blocked the production of inflammatory cytokines.

A study published by Serbian researchers in June 2009 in the journal *Clinical Nutrition* showed that olive leaf extract has a beneficial effect on rodents induced with experimental autoimmune encephalomyelitis (EAE), an animal model of brain inflammation. The researchers were drawn to testing olive leaf extract because there are fewer patients with multiple sclerosis in southern Europe, where the Mediterranean diet is prevalent. Because the benefits of olive oil have been examined extensively, this team of scientists wanted to also look at the compounds in olive leaf extract.

In a study published in *Biochemical Pharmacology* in 2010, a group of scientists in Spain tested oleanolic acid, a phytochemical found in olives and olive leaves, on mice with EAE. Their research showed that treatment with oleanolic acid before or at the onset of EAE improved neurological symptoms. They concluded that the oleanolic acid reduced the leakage of blood into brain cells and could lower the infiltration of inflammatory cells into the central nervous system.

Obesity

Obesity is a growing problem in nearly all industrialized nations, but it's especially prevalent in the United States, where there is excessive consumption of processed foods, refined sugars, and fast foods. Medical practitioners have begun to advocate prevention, which includes eating more plant-based foods and fewer animal products and getting at least thirty minutes of exercise or physical activity a day. These lifestyle changes have been shown to help prevent the numerous debilitating, persistent diseases associated with obesity.

Antioxidants are valuable in obesity prevention. An obese body develops chronic conditions, such as poor blood sugar control, high cholesterol, high blood pressure, and abdominal fat. This cluster of risk factors is referred to as metabolic syndrome. The American Heart Association estimates that about 34 percent of Americans are afflicted with metabolic syndrome.

When metabolism is affected, cells are affected, so it makes sense that antioxidants, which prevent or help reverse injury to cells, would counter some of the damage caused by obesity. Scientists have found that ingesting foods and plants rich in antioxidant compounds, such as dark chocolate, green and black teas, and olive leaf extract, is a natural way to achieve the same positive effects provided by antioxidant supplements.

The *Journal of Nutrition* published a study from The University of Queensland in Brisbane, Australia, that showed that olive leaf extract could reverse metabolic syndrome in rats. The scientists, inspired by what is known about the Mediterranean diet, wondered whether olive leaves would have the same effects as olive oil but without the fatty acid present in the oil. They used four groups of rats: one group was fed cornstarch and the other group was fed a high-fat, high-carbohydrate diet. They then divided those two groups and added olive leaf extract to half the diets of half the rats from each group. The rats on the high-fat, high-carbohydrate diet developed signs of metabolic syndrome. The rats with olive leaf extract added to their diet showed improved or normalized cardiovascular and metabolic signs; their hearts and livers were able to handle the fat and sugar better with the help of the antioxidants in olive leaf extract. It's not clear whether what works for rats would work for humans, but the results of studies like this are promising and prompt further investigation into human therapies.

Olive oil is also a healthy choice for anyone hoping to avoid metabolic syndrome or other health problems related to obesity. Consumed throughout the Mediterranean region, olive oil is a monounsaturated fat. Monounsaturated fats are most often found in plant foods as opposed to the saturated fats prevalent in animal-based foods, such as meat and dairy products. The healthy fats in olive oil can help lower LDL ("bad") cholesterol levels, especially when the oil is part of a diet and lifestyle that includes a high proportion of fruits and vegetables and regular exercise, both of which are also associated with the Mediterranean diet.

Osteoporosis

Bones are in a continuous state of transformation: new bone is forming as old bone tissue breaks down. As the body ages, bone mass is lost at a faster rate than it's gained. When the body loses too much bone or can't make enough new bone tissue, the result is osteoporosis. Although both men and women are affected by osteoporosis, postmenopausal women are especially susceptible to it. The World Health Organization (WHO) states that it's difficult to determine the worldwide incidence of osteoporosis because of variances in definitions and diagnoses, but looking at fracture rates can provide a sense of where the disease is most prevalent. According to the WHO website, Caucasian women living in temperate climates experience the most hip fractures. The rate of fractures is somewhat lower in women from Mediterranean and Asian countries, and women in Africa experience the fewest. Research is still being conducted on why rates are lower in these countries and how diet might play a part in the statistics.

Antioxidants likely have a role in osteoporosis. Antioxidants are naturally present in our bodies, but as we age, the ability to produce them slows down. At the same time—around the time that gray hairs start to appear—bone density begins to decline. The Western diet, loaded with animal fats and processed foods, accelerates the loss of bone mass. As they're metabolized, grains and animal proteins create an acid load in the body. To compensate, the body takes minerals and salt from the bones to neutralize the acid. A diet rich in alkalizing fruits and vegetables decreases the acid load, and the antioxidants in these foods help reduce the incidence of inflammation, which if gone unchecked, can eat away at bone health.

A team of scientists at the Tokyo Institute of Technology analyzed three of the compounds found in olives and olive leaves—oleuropein, hydroxytyrosol, and tyrosol—to determine their effectiveness on bone formation and bone loss. They tested cultured osteoblasts, which are cells that aid in bone formation, and osteoclasts, which are cells that weaken bones, on female mice with their ovaries removed. The oleuropein and hydroxytyrosol inhibited the formation of osteoclasts and suppressed the bone loss in the mice.

The study, which was published in the *European Journal of Pharmacology* in 2011, concluded that the olive polyphenols oleuropein and hydroxytyrosol may affect the formation and maintenance of bone and can be considered as remedies in the treatment of osteoporosis symptoms.

Olive Leaf Products

A search for olive leaf extract and other olive leaf products can result in a chorus of claims about oleuropein concentration or the concentration of other related compounds. Concentration of any one element in olive leaf extract shouldn't matter greatly, as long as the product is made from the whole leaves. Be aware that production isn't limited to the Mediterranean region; there are top-rated products and extracts from Australia, New Zealand, and the United States.

When choosing a product, one of the primary considerations to bear in mind is palatability. The main bioactive compound in olive leaves is oleuropein, which is the same bioactive compound that gives olives their bitter taste. Consequently, teas and liquid extracts will retain some of that bitterness. While some people enjoy the bitter taste, others prefer to bypass it. This can be a drawback of tinctures, especially if they are going to be used long term. However, their strong and fairly bitter taste can be minimized by mixing them with a little honey or fruit juice, or the unflavored liquid extract could be taken with food. A benefit of making olive leaf tea is that it can be sweetened, flavored with cinnamon or other spices, or mixed with flavorful teas, such as peppermint.

Other considerations when purchasing olive leaf products are convenience, quality, reliability, and consistency. Olive leaves and olive leaf extract come in several different forms: capsules, ethanolic tinctures, water/glycerine extracts (which may also be called tinctures), powder, or tea. It can be confusing trying to decide which product to choose. The following descriptions should help you determine which form is best for your needs.

As with any supplement, follow package instructions and consult a health care practitioner to discuss possible interactions with other medications.

Capsules

Some brands of olive leaf capsules contain liquid olive leaf extract. Other brands contain dried olive leaves, concentrated powdered extracts of olive leaves, or a combination of both. Capsules with the dried leaves or powdered extracts may also include excipients, which are nonactive ingredients added to the capsules' contents to increase bulk or prevent the machinery used to fill the capsules from clogging. Although most excipients are harmless, many natural health practitioners recommend avoiding certain ones, such as magnesium stearate, talc, and titanium dioxide.

A number of manufacturers state that olive leaf capsules contain more of the leaves' bioactive ingredients per dose than either tinctures or teas. For example, some claim that a 500 milligram capsule containing pure olive leaf extract standardized to 20 percent oleuropein will contain more oleuropein than a comparable dose of even a highly concentrated tincture or tea. Whether or not that is true, capsules are generally standardized, meaning that they will supply the same amount of oleuropein from capsule to capsule and from batch to batch. Most capsules have a maximum shelf life of about two years, as long as they are kept dry, cool, and out of direct sunlight. And capsules are convenient and easily transportable. Compared to other forms of olive leaf products, capsules are generally less expensive for the amount of oleuropein obtained.

Capsules that contain dried olive leaves combined with concentrated powdered olive leaf extract tend to be gentler and cause less stomach irritation. They also tend to provide a better balance of active ingredients. For a higher-quality product, seek out capsules with organic olive leaves.

Tinctures

Ethanolic tinctures, normally referred to just as tinctures, are liquids based on ethyl alcohol. Ethyl alcohol (drinking alcohol), usually derived from grains or cane sugar, is used to draw out the active ingredients from the leaves. An ethanol content between 30 and 40 percent is suitable for liquid tinctures of olive leaf extract. Although some people avoid the use of alcohol, it is considered a safe, practical, natural, and efficient medium for extracting and preserving the plant chemicals dissolved in it and delivering them into the bloodstream.

Olive leaf tinctures are absorbed rapidly through the mucous membranes of the mouth, stomach, and the first section of the small intestine. Because they are absorbed so quickly, tinctures are usually used for acute conditions––those that have a rapid onset and short duration. With their fast-acting capabilities, tinctures are effective for stopping early stages of viral and bacterial infections, especially in the upper respiratory tract and gut. They are also excellent for oral ulcers and infections. Most of the experimentation and clinical trials on blood pressure and other cardiovascular problems have been done using tinctures.

The efficient absorption of olive leaf tinctures makes dosing more accurate, as little or none of the bioactive ingredient is lost in the gut. Even though they may not contain as much oleuropein per dose as a few capsules, the superior absorption rate compensates for this. Nevertheless, good-quality tinctures tend to be more expensive than capsules due to the extraction time required and the higher cost of packaging and transporting flammable liquids.

Ethanolic tinctures are typically preferred by most herbalists and practitioners of natural medicine because they are versatile and can be mixed with other herbal tinctures for specific needs. Tinctures can be made from freshly picked olive leaves, thereby retaining the volatile substances that are lost in dried preparations. In addition, the extraction process is cold, which better protects some of the heat-sensitive polyphenols that would otherwise be damaged or destroyed in the drying process. Olive leaf tinctures require no additives, fillers, or preservatives. Virtually all compounds in the leaf are soluble in both water and ethanol, but many are more stable in solutions containing alcohol. Tinctures can be easily dispensed and administered in small or large doses for children or adults.

When purchasing tinctures, look for a clearly designated strength. The oleuropein in a tincture is almost twice as effective as the same quantity in capsule form. Seek out a product made with organic leaves grown by the manufacturer. Shelf life for a good-quality tincture is at least five years.

Water/Glycerine Extracts

Water/glycerine (glycerol) extracts are good general olive leaf tonics and contain no ethyl alcohol. These are generally marketed for antioxidant and immune support and cardiovascular health. Because they are alcohol-free, they are a popular choice for children or for general family use. Seek out products made from good-quality leaves; suppliers of high-quality leaves will promote this in their advertising material and product literature. Also look for standardized products that are certified to contain a specified percentage of oleuropein.

There are a few different extraction methods used, resulting in a range in the quality of products. The quality of olive leaf extract liquid is largely determined by the care taken in the extraction process, which can often be established from the information supplied by the manufacturer.

One method entails using fresh leaves that are cold pressed. This is considered the best method because only purified water is used to extract and dissolve the phytochemicals, retaining the volatile constituents of the leaf and causing no heat damage to them. Glycerol is then added as a preservative against opportunistic organisms, and natural flavorings are added to minimize the bitter taste of the olive leaves.

Another method entails using the dried leaves, which are chopped or crushed and soaked in a glycerol solution to extract the phytochemicals. This is a slower process because glycerol is a weak solvent. The process can be accelerated by heating the mixture, but that may cause some of the volatile constituents to become lost or damaged by the heat.

A stronger ethanol-free olive leaf extract liquid can be obtained by means of a normal ethanolic extraction followed by the removal of the ethanol by distillation in a partial vacuum; however, this can result in the unwanted removal of some of the volatile compounds. Other solvents, such as apple cider vinegar, may be used in the extraction process.

The advantages of water/glycerine extracts are that they are alcohol-free (for those who prefer that) and are generally milder, making them suitable for long-term supplementation and for children. Plus, they don't need additional preservatives, fillers, or excipients. However, the extraction process is not as efficient or comprehensive as cold ethanolic extraction. Oleuropein and many other plant substances are more stable in an alcohol solution than in water/glycerine, giving them a longer shelf life. In addition, water/glycerine extracts do not have as rapid or possibly as comprehensive absorption into the body as alcohol-based tinctures.

Powder

Ready-made olive leaf powder can be sprinkled on food, added to smoothies, mixed in juice, or even added to or made into an herbal tea. You can also use it to fill your own capsules and ensure they contain no undesirable fillers. When the powder is sprinkled on food or mixed in juice or smoothies, the taste will be masked, making it more palatable.

Most olive leaf powder is made simply from finely ground dried olive leaves, so it's not highly concentrated. But olive leaf standardized extract powder is made from a liquid extract of olive leaves that has been freeze-dried to a concentrated powder. It's available in a variety of strengths, indicated by the percentage of oleuropein the powdered extract contains. Typical concentrations range from 6 to 20 percent, and the cost will vary accordingly. Because these powders have a standardized strength, they are highly suitable for putting into capsules. Be aware, however, that while the highly concentrated olive leaf extract powders contain high levels of oleuropein, they may have lost other important constituents during the freeze-drying process. To ensure a broader range of constituents, mix them with high-quality powdered olive leaves (not an extract).

Tea

Although boiling destroys some of the volatile constituents, olive leaf tea provides most of the health benefits of olive leaf extract but in a gentler and more palatable way. An ideal replacement for common black tea, olive leaf tea contains no caffeine. It is said to be relaxing in standard concentrations and energy boosting in strong concentrations. In theory it should benefit the cardiovascular system in the same way that olive leaf extract does.

Although fairly well absorbed, concentrations of the olive leaf's active ingredients are low in the tea and results can typically take a few weeks. If the tea is made stronger for medicinal purposes, it will have a bitter taste. It can be made into iced tea with lemon and sweetener or added to ginger ale or soda water to mask the taste if desired.

Look for tea made from high-quality organic olive leaves. The leaves should be dried below 150 degrees F for the constituents to be fully active and effective. If you have access to olive trees, you can make your own tea from the leaves. Pick healthy, dry, unblemished leaves. Dry them in the oven at 150 degrees F. Tests have shown that more active ingredients are lost and more oxidative damage is incurred via air drying or sun drying than oven drying. After the leaves are dried, crush them by hand, remove the stalks, and put crushed leaves in paper packets or unbleached muslin tea bags for storage. Make tea as you normally would, using about 1 teaspoon of leaves per cup of water.

Side Effects and Contraindications

The Jarisch-Herxheimer reaction, or often just Herxheimer reaction, is a phenomenon that occurs when the body tries to eliminate toxins at a faster rate than they can be properly disposed of. It was first observed by German physician Karl Herxheimer and Australian physician Adolf Jarisch while they were treating syphilis patients. Jarisch recorded his observations in 1895; Herxheimer recorded his in 1902.

Also known as a "die-off," a Herxheimer reaction can entail a variety of responses. Here are some of the symptoms commonly experienced:

- Bloating and gas
- Chills
- Constipation
- Diarrhea
- Dizziness
- Elevated heart rate
- Fatigue
- Fever
- Headache
- Hives or rash
- Itchiness
- Joint or muscle pain
- Nausea
- Skin breakouts
- Sweating
- Swollen glands

Antibiotics can cause a Herxheimer reaction. Patients may experience the phenomenon when they're being treated for candida, Lyme disease, or rheumatoid arthritis. Olive leaf extract can cause a Herxheimer reaction too, because of its antimicrobial properties. Drinking plenty of water can help flush away the toxins and minimize symptoms. If the symptoms persist or make you too uncomfortable, lower the dosage or stop taking olive leaf extract.

Most people who aren't allergic to olives or olive tree pollen tolerate olive leaf extract quite well. However, olive leaf extract could potentially lower blood sugar, so taking olive leaf extract along with diabetes medication might cause glucose levels to drop too much. Olive products also seem to decrease blood pressure, so taking olive leaf extract with antihypertensive medications might cause blood pressure to fall too low.

Health and Beauty

If you've browsed the beauty products in any department store or drugstore, you may have noticed a surge in active ingredients such as plant peptides, plant stem cells, and antioxidants, and even a few nonplant active ingredients such as glycolic acid and copper. Products that merge cosmetics with pharmaceutical or medicinal ingredients are called cosmeceuticals. As they become more popular, these kinds of ingredients enter laboratories and end up in the jars and bottles of products we use at home. Board-certified dermatologist Nicholas Perricone, considered the father of cosmeceuticals, launched the theory that chronic inflammation speeds up the aging process, causing wrinkles and sagging skin. Perricone asserts that by treating inflammation the signs of aging will slow down. His approach covers not only using skin-care products that contain plant antioxidants but also changing the diet to include more high-antioxidant plant foods and fewer starchy and fatty foods.

Olive leaf extract, known for its antioxidant properties, appears as an ingredient in many beauty products. Olive leaves can also moisturize and cleanse the skin. Among the benefits attributed to topically applied olive leaf extract is a reduction in skin damage caused by UVB radiation. In addition, studies done with dry olive leaf extract show that it holds promise for preventing or treating skin cancer, including melanoma.

The antibacterial and anti-inflammatory properties of olive leaf extract are making it a rising star in acne treatments. Several skin-care lines have produced acne products containing olive leaf extract, from face washes to moisturizers to spot eliminators. There are anecdotal reports that powdered olive leaf extract can be made into a tincture and applied directly to problem skin, either as a stand-alone treatment or in combination with oral olive leaf extract.

Olive leaves are also showing up in fragrances. The scent of olive leaves can freshen a room by way of an oil diffuser, candle, or spray.

Suppliers

The following manufacturers make top-quality olive leaf products and sell directly to the public:

East Park Research

eastparkresearch.com

East Park Research sells a patented d-Lenolate form of olive leaf extract, made using a unique process that involves separating compounds derived from the leaves. The company also sells hair and skin care products with d-Lenolate.

Certified Nutraceuticals

certifiednutra.com

Certified Nutraceuticals has developed a supplement called Olea 25 that boasts a high percentage of hydroxytyrosol.

Olivus

olivus.com

Olivus offers a wide range of high-quality olive leaf supplements, including tincture, powder, capsules, and tea, as well as skin care products. Many products are certified organic, capsules contain no fillers, and the olive leaf is sourced from Mediterranean and California growers.

Other Recommended Brands

The following brands of high-quality olive leaf products are available through a variety of online retailers:

Barlean's
Gaia
L.A. Naturals
Life-Flo
Nature's Answer OleoPein Olive Leaf Alcohol-Free
Nature's Way
Seagate

References

Arts, I. C., D. R. Jacobs, M. Gross, L. J. Hamack, and A. R. Folsom. 2002. "Dietary Catechins and Cancer Incidence among Postmenopausal Women: The Iowa Women's Health Study (United States)." *Cancer Causes & Controls* 13 (4): 373–382. ncbi.nlm.nih.gov/pubmed/12074507.

Balch, Phyllis A. 2010. *Prescription for Nutritional Healing, Fifth Edition.* New York: Avery/Penguin.

Bisignano, G., A. Tomaino, R. Lo Cascio, G. Crisafi, N. Uccella, and A. Saija. 1999. "On the In-Vitro Antimicrobial Activity of Oleuropein and Hydroxytyrosol." *Journal of Pharmacy and Pharmacology* 51 (8): 971-974. ncbi.nlm.nih.gov/pubmed/10504039.

"The Compound in the Mediterranean Diet that Makes Cancer Cells 'Mortal.'" Research and Innovations Communication, The Ohio State University, last modified May 20, 2013, accessed March 3, 2015. http://researchnews.osu.edu/archive/apigenin.htm.

de Bock, M., J. Derraik, C. Brennan, J. Biggs, P. Morgan, S. Hodgkinson, P. Hofman, W. Cutfield. 2013. "Olive (Olea Europaea L.) Leaf Polyphenols Improve Insulin Sensitivity in Middle-Aged Overweight Men: A Randomized, Placebo-Controlled Crossover Trial." *PLOS ONE* 8 (3). http://journals.plos.org/plosone/article?id=10.1371/journal.pone.0057622.

Estruch, R., et al. 2013. "Primary Prevention of Cardiovascular Disease with a Mediterranean Diet." *New England Journal of Medicine* 368:1279–1290. nejm.org/doi/full/10.1056/NEJMoa1200303.

Flemmig J., K. Kuchta, J. Arnhold, and H. W. Rauwald. May 15, 2011. "*Olea Europaea* Leaf (ph.eur.) Extract as Well as Several of Its Isolated Phenolics Inhibit the Gout-Related Enzyme Xanthine Oxidase." *Phytomedicine* 18 (7): 561–6.

Frankel, E. N., J. B. German, J. E. Kinsella, E. Parks, and J. Kanner. 1993. "Inhibition of Oxidation of Human Low-Density Lipoprotein by Phenolic Substances in Red Wine." *The Lancet* 341 (8843): 454–457. thelancet.com/journals/lancet/article/PII0140-6736(93)90206-V/abstract.

Garcia-Villalba, R., M. Larrosa, S. Possemiers, F. A. Tomas-Barberan, and J. C. Espin. 2013. "Bioavailability of Phenolics From an Oleuropein-Rich Olive (Olea Europaea) Leaf Extract and Its Acute Effect on Plasma Antioxidant Status: Comparison Between Pre- and Postmenopausal Women." *European Journal of Nutrition* 53 (4): 1015–1027. ncbi.nlm.nih.gov/pubmed/24158653.

Gong D, C. Geng, L. Jiang, L. Wang, H. Yoshimura, and L. Zhong. March 2012. "Mechanisms of Olive Leaf Extract-Ameliorated Rat Arthritis Caused by Kaolin and Carrageenan." *Phytother Res* 26 (3): 397–402.

Hagiwara, K., T. Goto, M. Araki, H. Miyazaki, and H. Hagiwara. 2011. "Olive Polyphenol Hydroxytyrosol Prevents Bone Loss." *European Journal of Pharmacology* 665 (1–3): 78-84. sciencedirect.com/science/article/pii/S0014299911004134.

Impellizzeri D, E. Esposito, E. Mazzon, et al. December 2011. "Oleuropein Aglycone, an Olive Oil Compound, Ameliorates Development of Arthritis Caused by Injection of Collagen Type II in Mice." *J Pharmacol Exp Ther* 339 (3): 859–69.

Kilham, Chris. "The Healing Power of Olive Leaf." Foxnews.com, January 23, 2013. foxnews.com/health/2013/01/23/healing-power-olive-leaf/.

Kimura, Y., and M. Sumiyoshi. 2009. "Olive Leaf Extract and Its Main Component Oleuropein Prevent Chronic Ultraviolet B Radiation-Induced Skin Damage and Carcinogenesis in Hairless Mice." *Journal of Nutrition* 139 (11): 2079–2086. http://jn.nutrition.org/content/139/11/2079.long.

Kumamoto, Carol. 2011. "Inflammation and Gastrointestinal *Candida* Colonization." *Current Opinion in Microbiology* 14 (4): 386–391. ncbi.nlm.nih.gov/pmc/articles/PMC3163673/

Lim, D., H. Cho, J. Kim, C. Nho, K. Lee, and J. Park. January 2012. "Luteolin decreases IGF-II production and downregulates insulin-like growth factor-I receptor signaling in HT-29 human colon cancer cells." *BMC Gastroenterology* 12:9. biomedcentral.com/1471–230X/12/9.

Markin, D., L. Duek, and I. Berdicevsky. 2003. "In Vitro Antimicrobial Activity of Olive Leaves." Mycoses 46 (3–4): 132–136. http://onlinelibrary.wiley.com/enhanced/doi/10.1046/j.1439-0507.2003.00859.x/.

Martin, Jeanne Marie, and Zoltan Rona. 2000. *Complete Candida Yeast Guidebook, Revised 2nd Edition.* New York: Three Rivers Press.

Martin, R., J. Carvalho-Tavares, M. Hernandez, M. Arnes, V. Ruiz-Gutierrez, and M. L. Nieto. 2010. "Beneficial Actions of Oleanolic Acid in an Experimental Model of Multiple Sclerosis: A Potential Therapeutic Role." *Biochemical Pharmacology* 79 (2): 198–208. ncbi.nlm.nih.gov/pubmed/19679109.

Mijatovic, S. A., G. Timotijevic, D. Milijkovic, J. Radovic, D. Maksimovic-Ivanic, D. Dekanski, S. Stosic-Grujicic. 2011. "Multiple Antimelanoma Potential of Dry Olive Leaf Extract." *International Journal of Cancer* 128 (8): 1955–1965. ncbi.nlm.nih.gov/pubmed/20568104.

Miljkovic, D., D. Dekanski, Z. Miljkovic, M. Momcilovic, and M. Mostarica-Stojkovic. 2009. "Dry Olive Leaf Extract Ameliorates Experimental Autoimmune Encephalomyelitis." *Clinical Nutrition* 28 (3): 346–350. ncbi.nlm.nih.gov/pubmed/19386399.

"Nutrition Health Topics 5: Population Nutrient Intake Goals for Preventing Diet-Related Chronic Diseases," World Health Organization, who.int/nutrition/topics/5_population_nutrient/en/ (accessed March 4, 2015).

Perrinjaquet-Moccetti, T., A. Busjahn, C. Schmidlin, C. Schmidt, B. Bradi, C. Aydogan. 2008. "Food Supplementation with an Olive (Olea Europaea L.) Leaf Extract Reduces Blood Pressure in Borderline Hypertensive Monozygotic Twins." *Phytotherapy Research* 22 (9): 1239–1242. ncbi.nlm.nih.gov/pubmed/18729245.

Pollan, Michael. 2008. *In Defense of Food: An Eater's Manifesto.* New York: Penguin.

Pollan, Michael. May 15, 2013. "Some of My Best Friends Are Germs." *The New York Times Magazine.*

Poudyal, H., F. Campbell, and L. Brown. 2010. "Olive Leaf Extract Attenuates Cardiac, Hepatic, and Metabolic Changes in High-Carbohydrate-, High-Fat Fed Rats." *Journal of Nutrition* 140 (5): 946-953. http://jn.nutrition.org/content/140/5/946.full.

Somova, L., F. O. Shode, P. Ramnanan, A. Nadar. 2003. "Antihypertensive, Antiatherosclerotic and Antioxidant Activity of Triterpenoids Isolated from *Olea Europaea*, Subspecies *Africana* Leaves." *Journal of Ethnophar macology* 84 (2–3): 299–305. ncbi.nlm.nih.gov/pubmed/12648829.

Taddonio, Patrice. March 6, 2005. "Unexpected Discoveries," Profile: Pathogen-Host Research. TuftsNow newsletter, Tufts University. tufts.edu/home/feature/?p=pathogens&p3=3 (accessed March 17, 2015).

Takeda, R., T. Koike, I. Taniguchi, and K. Tanaka. 2013. "Double-Blind Placebo-Controlled Trial of Hydroxytyrosol of Olea Europaea on Pain in Gonarthrosis." *Phytomedicine* 20 (10): 861-864. ncbi.nlm.nih.gov/pubmed/23746949.

Wojcikowski, K., L. Stevenson, D. Leach, H. Wohlmuth, and G. Gobe. 2007. "Antioxidant Capacity of 55 Medicinal Herbs Traditionally Used to Treat the Urinary System: A Comparison Using a Sequential Three-Solvent Extraction Process." *Journal of Alternative and Complementary Medicine* 13 (1): 103-110. ncbi.nlm.nih.gov/pubmed/17309384.

About the Author

Lori Barrett is a freelance writer living in Chicago. Her writing has appeared in the *Wall Street Journal*, *Notre Dame Magazine*, *Time Out Chicago*, and *The Fourth River*. She became interested in nutrition and health after her son, at the age of eight, decided to become a vegetarian.